GET STRONGER, LIVE LONGER

500 Affirmations for Optimal Health,
Rapid Healing, and Maximum Longevity

Stan Munslow
4G Publishing

Get Stronger, Live Longer
500 Affirmations for Optimal Health,
Rapid Healing, and Maximum Longevity

© 2018 by Stan Munslow
4G Publishing
Coventry, Rhode Island U.S.A.

ISBN-13: 978-1987557572
ISBN-10: 1987557573

All rights reserved under the International and Pan-American Copyright Conventions. No part of this book may be reproduced or transmitted in any form or by any means, electronic or mechanical, including photocopying, recording, or by any information storage and retrieval system, without permission in writing from the publisher.

IMPORTANT NOTICE

The information provided in this book is designed to provide helpful information on the subjects discussed. This book is not meant to be used, nor should it be used, to diagnose or treat any medical condition. For diagnosis or treatment of any medical problem, consult your own physician. The publisher and author are not responsible for any specific health or allergy needs that may require medical supervision and are not liable for any damages or negative consequences from any treatment, action, application or preparation, to any person reading or following the information in this book.

For life.

INTRODUCTION

"I know that I look, feel, and behave several decades younger than my actual age, and much of that is because I believe you are what you think you are. This is called positive affirmation, and it's a really strong tool."

Joan Collins

It's true! You *are* what you think you are. Your body *is* what you think it to be. Your health *is* as good as you say it is. Your habitual thoughts, beliefs, and statements about your body have an almost unbelievably strong impact upon your health, your ability to heal from illness or surgery, and your prospects for living a very long life.

For good or bad.

If your thoughts, beliefs, and statements about your health lie mostly in the negative, the disempowering, or even the destructive categories, your body *will* listen. And somehow, at some time, these statements will likely manifest in your body in the form of chronic or frequent illness, poor prospects for healing and recovery, and most likely less-than-admirable odds on making it beyond the coveted and seemingly elusive century mark.

The good news is that the opposite is every bit as true. If you feed your body a steady diet of deliberately healthful, empowering, and positive thoughts, beliefs, and statements, your body *will* listen. And it will respond accordingly.

And if you send your body messages in the form of powerful and positive statements—*which you repeat emphatically and often*—the trillions of cells that make up your body will really sit up and take notice!

These statements, good or bad, are referred to as *affirmations*. And that's what this book is all about. Affirmations—in this case, affirmations of the positive kind—affirmations of the positive and very powerful kind:

Five hundred powerful affirmations that will help set you on a direct path toward optimal health, rapid healing, and maximum longevity.

The use of positive affirmation is very widespread among people from all walks of life—from Olympic athletes to rock stars to top CEOs. They are widespread because affirmations are very powerful and effective in bringing about desired outcomes.

What's even more astounding is that, if the use of affirmations is so effective in acting upon *outside* circumstances, such as the generation of wealth or success, just imagine what they can do for your own physiology!

Most people are well aware of the mind-body connection. However, thanks to the astonishing discoveries made in the field of quantum physics, we now know that this connection is even more profound than most people ever realized—far more profound. As you will learn, your mind doesn't just affect or control your body, it literally creates it!

Read those words again:

Your mind doesn't just affect or control your body, it literally creates it!

This means that the beliefs you hold about your body—and the repeated messages you send it—have a significant impact upon your well-being. And the five hundred affirmations presented in this book will begin to feed your mind-body the very messages it needs most in order to remain in excellent health for a very long time.

Don't worry if you don't believe some of these statements at first. Just allow the words to repeatedly seep into your subconscious. In time, you will come to see that your health, well-being, and longevity really are in your hands far, far more than you could ever have imagined. Affirmations work. Affirmations work wonders. And now you are about to discover the very best affirmations your body could ever know.

This book is divided into three parts. In the first: *Affirm Your Good Health*, you will discover an entirely new way of looking at your body which will begin to put you in far greater control of its inner goings-on and ultimately give it a whole new lease on life.

In part two: *Affirm Your Rapid Healing*, you will learn powerful new ways to more quickly and more easily recover from illness, injury, and surgery. Taken to its fullest, you may even find that supposedly "incurable" diseases can be, and already have been, cured by many individuals — using nothing but the power of positive affirmation.

Finally, in part three: *Affirm Your Longevity*, you will learn the best ways to think and act that will help to add years — healthy, vital years — to your lifespan. You'll be learning attitudes, actions, and daily habits from many of the world's oldest people and, like them, you may quite possibly extend your lifespan beyond one hundred years.

Please note, however, that this book is not a substitute for professional health care — it is a supplement to it. And while it makes no promises or guarantees, you are most certainly doing the right thing for your body and your well-being by infusing the following affirmations into your mind, body, and spirit.

Furthermore, please understand that, by coming to believe these affirmations, you are seeking, more than anything else, to improve your health or to more quickly recover from illness or surgery. You are not necessarily going to cause every statement you make to come true all the time. Affirming "I do not get sick" doesn't necessarily mean that you will never get sick (although it could); it means that, at the very least, you are helping yourself to not get sick as often. And that is, ahem, nothing to sneeze at!

Read this book often. Allow the health-enhancing statements to seep deep down into your mind and ultimately become part of your new paradigm on health, healing, and longevity. Better yet, record them (perhaps enlisting the help of your loved ones, whose voices you love most!) for listening when you are going to bed or driving in your car.

You are giving your body an amazing gift by reading, repeating, and absorbing the affirmations in this book. May they provide you with the wisdom to achieve optimal health, the strength to enjoy rapid recovery from illness or surgery, and the tools you need to live a very long life!

Part One
AFFIRM YOUR GOOD HEALTH

"Our body is shaped by our mind, for we become what we think."

Buddha

Thrive with Awareness and Understanding

The first step in achieving optimal health is to understand the true *depth* of the mind-body connection. Thanks to discoveries in the field of quantum physics, we are coming to understand that our thoughts not only affect the body ... that our thoughts not only control the body ... but that our thoughts—to an almost unfathomable degree—actually and literally *create* the body.

Read the following affirmations silently or aloud—with conviction and feeling:

1

My body is made of cells—my cells, like all matter, are made of vibrating bundles of *energy*. All matter—all things—are made of energy.
My body is made of energy.

2

Energy, according to quantum science, is made of awareness—of *intelligence*. In truth, my
body is made of intelligence.

3
My intelligence controls and creates my body —
whether I'm aware of it or not.

4
My mind creates my body. My thoughts, beliefs,
opinions, and expectations literally
create my body.

5
My thinking creates the very cells of my body.

6
I am literally what I think.

7
For good or bad, my body is what I
continually think it to be.

8
My body is created by my thoughts about it.

9
My health is made good or bad by my
habitual thinking.

10

I think my body and my health into existence — and I understand that this truth is based on hard science.

11

My health responds to my thoughts and beliefs about it — just as it always has.

12

We are what we think — I *am* what I *think*. I think health, strength, energy — therefore, I *am* healthy, strong and energetic.

13

I think only the best thoughts in regard to my body.

14

I think health and well-being — always. And I will have them.

15

I think strength and vitality — always. And I will have them.

16

I think youthfulness and vigor — always. And I will have them.

17
I steer my thinking away from fearful thoughts about "possible illness."

18
I don't anticipate illness. I don't expect to get sick. I continually anticipate good health — and I will have it.

19
If I shift my attention away from occasional and temporary aches, pains, and illnesses — and focus, instead, on good health — I will get more of the same — I will enjoy more good health.

20
If I shift my attention away from occasional and temporary aches, pains, and illnesses — and focus instead, on good health — I will have fewer aches, pains, and illnesses.

21
My body is healthy. My body is strong. My body is perfect.

22
My health largely responds to the positive nature of my thoughts about it.

23

I often visualize all the parts of my body as perfect — as functioning perfectly — whether they are at the present time or not. My body listens to my thoughts. I think ... I become.

24

I see my body not as it is "appears" to be, but as I *want* it to be. I understand that this is *the way* of highly successful individuals: to continually focus attention not on the way things are, but on the way we *want* them to be.

25

Next, I understand that nearly all the cells in my body will be replaced within seven years' time. My body is, on a cellular level, seven years old or less. It is ever-changing and ever renewed.

26

I am, to no small degree, ageless.

27

My body is less than seven years old.
I repeat this profound statement often.

28

My cells live, my cells die, my cells are replaced. They come and go. My body makes itself anew constantly. Knowing this keeps me feeling young.

29

Since most of the cells that make up my body are less than seven years old, I understand that there are now virtually no cells in my body that were "inherited" from my parents. The body I have now is *not* the same body I was born with.

30

I understand that the ability of genetics to influence health is highly overrated. But the ability of one's *thinking* to influence health is *highly underrated*.

31

Genetics "influence" my health to as large or as small a degree as I say they do.

32

Since there are virtually no cells in my body that were inherited from my parents, I refuse to expect that genetics will predetermine my health.

33
My *beliefs* about my body are a much stronger determiner of my health than luck, fate, or genetics.

34
My *health habits* are a much stronger determiner of my physical well-being than genetics.

35
My *expectations* are a much stronger determiner of my health than genetics.

36
My *positive thoughts* about my body create my very being — my very healthy being, for what I think, I become.

Thrive with a Positive Mental Attitude

The next step in maintaining good health is to infuse our thinking with positivity and our emotions with joy, exuberance, confidence, gratitude, enthusiasm and bliss—and, in so doing, create a body that is the physical and physiological manifestation of all these.

37
My continual and chosen feelings of *happiness* and *joy* help tremendously to create my robust and vital body.

38
My continual and chosen feelings of *enthusiasm* and *exuberance* help to create my healthy, strong body.

39
My laughter literally prevents and kills disease.

40
I laugh often and much.

41
In this life, I generally don't take things —
or myself — too seriously.

42
The cells of my body operate at peak performance
when they are infused with my positive, loving,
and cheerful thoughts and feelings.

43
Happiness and a positive outlook are *choices*. They
are decisions. And I choose to be happy.

44
I choose to live with joy and gratitude.

45
I choose to keep my disposition and my outlook
positive and upbeat.

46
I understand the power of *gratitude*. I understand that
the universe gives us more of that which we are
grateful for. I am, therefore, grateful for all the
good in my life, including my good health.

47
I am grateful for my life.

48
I am grateful for the miracle of my healthy body.

49
I give thanks for my strong, amazing heart.

50
I give thanks for my miraculous and capable mind.

51
I am grateful for my eyes and ears — for the gift of sight and hearing that is denied to so many.

52
I am grateful for my skilled and capable hands.

53
I am thankful for my hard-working lungs and vital organs.

54
I am thankful for my incredible and powerful immune system.

55
I am thankful for my strong bones and muscles.

56
I am grateful—truly grateful—for each and every part of my amazing and wonderful body and all that it does for me.

57
Every morning, I wake up and give thanks for the miracle of my healthy body.

58
Every morning, I give thanks for my excellent health.

59
Every morning, I give thanks for being alive another day.

60
Next, I understand the incredible power of *positive expectation*.

61
I tend to avoid illness because I *expect* to avoid illness.

62
I remain youthful and energetic because
I expect to remain youthful and energetic.

63
I remain healthy because I expect — and not merely
hope — to remain healthy. My body
responds in kind.

64
I expect only the best from my amazing body.

65
Next, I understand that *what we focus on, expands*.
Thus, I focus on unending good health.

66
I focus on my strong and perfect body.

67
When I have an illness, I keep my thoughts focused
on regaining perfect health, not on being sick.

68
The better my thoughts, the better my health.

69

My positive mental attitude has tremendous power in keeping me healthy — especially when I wholeheartedly believe in this power.

Stan Munslow

Thrive with Good Nutrition

We are what we eat — literally and completely. Looking at food from the point of view of creating our bodies, improving our health, and increasing our life expectancy, we come to realize how important good nutrition is and to choose the foods we eat with utmost care.

70
I am what I eat — I am literally what I eat.

71
What I eat is what I am.

72
My food isn't just inside me — it *is* me.

73
Good food doesn't just make me healthy, it makes *me*.

74
The food I eat creates my body. I choose what
I eat with utmost care.

75
I understand that every cell in my body is made
from something I've eaten during
the past seven years.

76
I eat mostly plants.

77
I eat foods high in protein, fiber, antioxidants,
and other beneficial nutrients.

78
I avoid sugar as much as I can, not only to improve
my dental health, but to help prevent cancer.

79
I cut down on fat and I avoid all trans-fats.

80
I steer clear of sodium.

81
To the greatest extent possible, I shun foods grown with GMOs (genetically modified organisms).

82
I avoid chemical additives. They are not necessary and have no place in my food — or in me.

83
I eat as much organic food as I can — chemical pesticides and optimum health are mutually exclusive.

84
I read labels and avoid foods containing harmful or non-nourishing ingredients as much as possible.

85
I eat only the most healthful food I can find, even if it costs more. I am worth the investment.

86
I avoid toxins such as pesticides, preservatives, artificial flavors, artificial colors, and other food additives as much as possible.

87
If I can't pronounce it, I don't eat it.

88
I educate myself by reading credible books and articles on the subject of nutrition and food safety.

89
Healthful food means a healthy me.

90
Healthful food *becomes* a healthy me.

91
I eat to create my body and to nourish my body — not for the sole purpose of momentarily entertaining my tongue.

92
My brain chooses the food I eat — not my taste buds, not my cravings, and not advertising.

93
I see food as nourishment first, pleasure second.

94
Food creates my body. I eat for creation, not recreation.

95
I *use* food, I don't glorify it and I don't obsess on it.

96
I have plenty of interests to make my life enjoyable and complete. Snacking, pigging out, and mindless eating need not be among them.

97
I eat only as much as I need in order to satisfy my hunger and nourish my irreplaceable body.

98
I fully understand and appreciate the importance of food in building my body and keeping it in top condition.

Thrive with Exercise

Exercise does so much for our bodies, minds, and souls. It makes us strong, gives us energy, helps us to achieve and maintain a healthy weight, strengthens our heart, fights depression, prevents illness, and much more. But we need not run marathons nor pump iron in order to enjoy its benefits. Light to moderate exercise, four or five days a week is all it takes.

99
I move my body every chance I get.

100
I crave movement.

101
I enjoy physical activity with all my heart.

102
Dancing, gardening, strolling, sports, bicycling —
I love moving my body in so many ways.

103
I choose to look forward to exercising my body each day.

104
I exercise at the same time each day in order to make it into a habit more quickly.

105
I am *not* one for sitting around for hours on end.

106
I prefer movement over stagnation.

107
I love to exercise!

108
I love being active!

109
I love feeling strong — and growing ever stronger.

110
I love the feeling — the high — brought on by the pleasure-inducing hormones known as endorphins, which exercise gives rise to.

111
I love the feeling of having more energy.

112
I love the feeling of having more muscle.

113
I love adding more years—stronger, healthier, more vital years—to my life through exercise.

114
I love knowing that, by exercising, I am doing something good for myself and my loved ones.

115
I don't discount the importance of rest, but I do discount the allure of living a sedentary lifestyle.

116
As the saying goes, I would much rather wear out than rust out.

117
Being chronically lazy is definitely not my style.

118
I walk whenever possible. I don't need to be "carried" by a car everywhere I go.

119
When running errands, I seek the farthest parking spot from the door.

120
For short trips, I walk or cycle whenever I can.

121
I opt for the stairs whenever I can.

122
I tend not to shun physical exertion — unless directed by a physician to do so.

123
Even while sitting on a sofa or at a desk, I use hand weights, I do isometric exercises, and I perform simple muscle flexes in my hands, arms, shoulders, abdomen, and legs.

124
Even while standing, I do gentle, little squats to power up my thighs.

125
Exercise makes me feel good — physically, mentally, and emotionally.

126
I am fit and active.

127
I am strong and vital.

128
I love keeping my body strong.

129
I love keeping my body active.

130
I love keeping my body going.

131
To me, "growing older" does not have to mean slowing down or growing weaker.

132
I value all the benefits of exercise.

133
Exercise keeps my mind, body, and spirit in top condition.

134
Exercise keeps me strong and trim.

135
Exercise clears my brain.

136
Exercise gives me more energy.

137
The benefits I receive from exercise are far too valuable to ignore or pass up.

Thrive with Stress Reduction

The bad news is that chronic stress can damage our health and render us more prone to illness. The good news is that stress is largely *avoidable* — and in more ways than we may realize.

138
I understand that stress is largely a matter of whether or not I *choose* to perceive a situation as stressful in the first place.

139
I understand that stress is largely a matter of *choice*.

140
I understand that it is often not the situation itself that is stressful, it is my *interpretation* of it.

141
I avoid most stress by choosing to regard most situations as simply *not* all that important.

142
I am grateful that, more often than not, I can choose acceptance and ease over stress and worry.

143
I understand that, in many seemingly stressful situations, taking three slow, deep breaths is all it takes to avoid stressing out.

144
I understand that many supposed stressors are, in fact, not that important and not worth stressing over. As author Richard Carlson so brilliantly said: "Don't sweat the small stuff — and it's all small stuff."

145
There are many situations in my day-to-day life which I can choose to regard as no big deal: traffic, computer glitches, bad-hair days, and so on.

146
I am finding it easier to laugh at misadventures which, before now, would have upset me.

147
To not stress out is my *choice*.

148
To not worry is my *decision*.

149
To choose a more enlightened and health-conscious response to a trying situation is *my right*.

150
I realize that, if I have no control over a situation, then worrying won't help. So, I choose not to worry about it and just get on with my life.

151
If, on the other hand, I *can* control or fix a situation, then worrying about it won't help either. I just fix it and get on with my life.

152
I am well aware that worrying never helps. Never ever. Acceptance does. Corrective action does.

153
The same goes for negative rumination. It does nothing but harm my physiology and darken my spirit; I avoid it as well.

154
I have better things to do with my brain than ruminating for hours on end on something that is over and done with.

155
I have better things to do with my precious time than ruminating on something that really wasn't even a big deal in the first place.

156
Likewise, I avoid playing the "blame game." I realize that it is toxic to my physical and emotional well-being.

157
Ditto for complaining. It does neither my mood, nor my physiology an ounce of good. I have no interest in that waste-of-energy either.

158
Overall, I have no interest in playing the role of "the victim."

159
I understand that prolonged depression is harmful to my overall health. I will seek counseling and ask my doctor about antidepressants if I should find myself depressed for any extended period of time.

160
I understand that, no matter how long I may live, my time on this planet is too short to waste with chronic worry, negativity, anger, fear, sadness, regret, or apprehension.

161
I choose instead to live a long, healthy, carefree, meaningful, loving, and joyful life.

162
I choose instead to live with happiness, gratitude, exuberance, and a positive mental attitude.

Thrive with a Healthful Lifestyle

To be healthy is to *live* healthy — to live in a manner that does right for our bodies and to make choices each day that promote our well-being and keep us from harm.

163
I live a very healthful and health-conscious lifestyle.

164
I avoid unnecessary threats to my well-being.

165
I avoid speeding and aggressive driving.

166
I avoid driving under the influence — whether that be under the influence of alcohol or texting.

167
I avoid excessive alcohol consumption.

168
I do not smoke and I avoid second-hand smoke as well, for it is just as dangerous as smoking itself.

169
I avoid taking unnecessary risks that jeopardize my health and well-being.

170
I don't live in fear, but I do live with care.

171
I avoid taxing my heart with excessive rushing, overwork, or an aggressive, intense, confrontational, over-driven personality.

172
No matter what my career, I don't overdo. I refuse to harm my physiology and potentially shorten my life in the name of making more money.

173
I tend to avoid trying to get through my days — and, thus, my life — faster.

174
I avoid a harsh, aggressive, competitive, time-obsessed, workaholic lifestyle in all its forms.

175

I trade pushy, bossy, negative, hot-tempered,
intolerant, and intense ... with calm,
cool, collected, wise, kind, gentle,
and even-keeled.

176

I practice some form of mind-body work, be
that yoga, Taiichi, or meditation.

177

I practice the art of mindfulness in all that I do. I give
whatever I'm doing — or whomever I'm
with — my full attention.

178

More and more, I engage in activities that
give me great pleasure.

179

I maintain a sense of *equanimity* — of calm,
non-judging steadiness of mind —
during trying situations.

180

I maintain calm by remembering to take several deep,
long breaths during difficult situations. I maintain
ease by practicing the fine art of acceptance.

181
I live in the present.

182
I live in the moment.

183
I live in the *now*. Now is, indeed, all I have.

184
I will continue to work on building a lifestyle that keeps my blood pressure down, my spirits up, and my body intact.

Thrive with Loving Connections

Maintaining loving connections with friends and family, as well as a sense of community with people around us, is so vital to our mental, emotional, and physiological well-being that entire books have been written on the subject. As much as possible, we need to put people first on our list of priorities and activities.

185
I understand that loving connection is very strongly linked to my health and well-being.

186
I value my family relationships.

187
I treasure my close friendships.

188
I put interaction with friends and family high on my list of priorities.

189
I work hard to maintain my friendships.

190
I put a premium on meeting new people and making new friends.

191
Being social is so important to my physical, mental, and emotional well-being, I simply ignore and overcome any trepidation I may have about meeting new people.

192
I understand that human interaction and connection extend beyond friendship to include people with whom I come in contact throughout my day.

193
I value my interactions with service personnel, neighbors, coworkers, passers-by, and folks near me in the checkout line.

194
I smile, give praise when it is due, and I look forward to brief exchanges with others, in part, for all the benefits they provide my mind, body, and soul.

195
I utilize the power of social media and the Internet at-large to provide me with an additional layer of connection with others.

196
I use technology, but I don't overuse or abuse it.

197
I use social media as a supplement to flesh-and-blood interaction, but not as a substitute for it.

198
I offer a warm, sincere smile to everyone I meet.

199
I understand that the process of smiling at others benefits me every bit as much as the recipient.

200
I understand that having a pet to cuddle—one who will offer me unconditional love in return—has been proven to lower my blood pressure and provide a host of other important health benefits.

201
I enjoy occasional periods of solitude, but I put a premium on being with others.

202
I love striking up conversations with just about anyone.

203
I enjoy being warm and friendly, and enjoying community with my fellow man and woman.

204
I am a people person.

205
I am loving.

206
I am lovable.

207
I greatly enjoy meeting new people and making new friends.

208
Friendships are good for my body as well as my soul.

209
I am warm and good-natured.

210
I am kind and pleasant.

211
I am personable and cordial.

212
I am friendly and sociable.

213
I am affable and amicable.

214
I am well-liked and well-respected.

215
I am a great listener.

216
I am welcoming and outgoing.

217
I am amiable and neighborly.

218
I am engaging and kind-hearted.

219
I value my close, loving relationships with the members of my family.

220
I am thankful for my loving relationships with the members of my family.

221
I give hugs freely.

222
I am affectionate.

223
I enjoy appropriate touching and being touched.

224
I value the importance of touch regarding my health and my emotional well-being.

225
I am empathetic and easygoing.

226
I empathize with others. I feel for them and I feel *with* them.

227
My spirit is buoyed and my physiology healed by frequent loving contact.

228
I understand that to love — deeply and unconditionally — is one of the most beneficial things I can do for my health and well-being.

229
I am healthy.

230
I am strong.

231
I am vital.

232
My body is in perfect health.

233
I love being alive!

234
Above all else, my good health is a *choice*.

Part Two

AFFIRM YOUR RAPID HEALING

"The natural healing force within each of us is the greatest force in getting well."

Hippocrates

The Power of Positive Energy

When it comes to healing from injury, recovering from illness, or bouncing back after surgery, positivity is the world's greatest elixir. Once again, our bodies are made from the energy of our thoughts and emotions. To keep this energy positive is vital. To think positively truly is a miracle cure.

235

I understand that, since my body is made of energy, when I infuse it continually with positive energy in the form of joy, humor, gratitude, and most of all, positive expectations, my healing is strengthened and accelerated.

236

Even when I have an illness occupying one part of my body, I continue to see the rest of my body as healthy.

237
To the greatest extent I can muster, I remain happy, upbeat, and full of positive energy throughout my illness, both to lessen its severity and shorten its duration.

238
Smiling is good for my physiology. No illness has the power to keep me from smiling.

239
No illness is stronger than my spirit.

240
I am fully aware that my positivity, happiness, and hope will help to mend my body to the extent that I believe in its power to do so.

241
When illness comes into my body, I focus my attention not on the illness, but on all the *good* that is in my life.

242
When illness comes into my body, I focus my attention not on the illness but on those parts of my body that remain healthy and unaffected by the illness.

243

When I am ill or recovering from surgery, I focus on *being well* — on the *feeling* of being well. As often as I can, I visualize being well, using all my senses and with deep emotion.

244

I understand that laughter really is the best medicine. Science has proven time and time again that laughter strengthens my immune system and helps to rid my body of disease.

245

Whenever I am sick, I watch funny movies and standup comics and literally laugh myself into a speedier recovery.

246

Whenever I am sick, I smile, I laugh, I think positive, uplifting thoughts and keep my mind off the sickness.

247

I am very well aware that my recovery from illness or surgery will be accelerated in proportion to how much happiness and positivity I can muster.

The Power of Strength

If and when an illness comes our way, we can choose to remain strong—strong-willed and strong minded—and in so doing, return strength to our physical body as well. Never regard your illness or ailment as being larger and more powerful than you. Never allow it to have that upper hand. Be confident, be strong, and never stop seeing yourself as the ultimate victor!

248
I am stronger than my illness.

249
I am tougher than my illness.

250
I am more powerful than the diseased cells taking up temporary residence inside me. Like healthy cells, diseased cells are, in fact, *my* cells. They belong to me and they are every bit as under my control as every other cell in my body.

251
I am strong, tough, and resilient.

252
I am more persistent than my illness.

253
I choose to remain mentally and emotionally strong.

254
I choose to call upon my inner strength in fighting this illness.

255
Acting from strength or weakness is always my choice. I choose to act from strength.

256
I've got a whole lot of fight inside me.

257
My body's immune system is tougher than my illness.

258
My immune system can easily kill any unwelcome germs or cells that come along.

259
My immune system is very powerful.

260
My spirit is unshakable and unbeatable.

261
My body is tough — if I say it is.

262
My soul is resilient — if I say it is.

263
My immune system is unbeatable — if I say it is.

264
When I am ill, I think thoughts of strength, power, tenacity, and victory.

265
I don't give in and I don't give up.

266

I give this fight everything I have — and I expect nothing short of triumph.

267

I choose to call upon all the inner strength I can muster in fighting my illness or my healing after surgery — and to reap all the rewards of an accelerated recovery and rapid healing.

The Power of
Positive Expectation

We don't always get what we want in life, we get what we *expect*—particularly that which we expect continually and with strong conviction. Since our bodies are created by our thoughts (including our expectations), this axiom goes doubly true in matters of healing and recovery. For good or bad, in health and healing, as with all else, we usually get what we expect.

268
I understand that to expect illness increases its likelihood and that to expect wellness increases its likelihood.

269
I understand that living in constant fear or expectation of getting sick increases its probability.

270
I understand the incredible power that my continually viewing my body as healthy has upon my physiology.

271
I don't get sick. Period.

272
I expect to remain healthy and disease free. I believe it to my core. Yes, I may be nonetheless stricken with illness on rare occasion, but these occurrences will be greatly diminished by my positive expectations of continued good health.

273
I expect to remain healthy and disease free. Yes, I may be nonetheless stricken with illness on rare occasion, but there will most likely be fewer of them and my recovery from these illnesses will be accelerated by my positive expectations.

274
If and when I have an illness, I completely expect a speedy recovery.

275
I expect — with conviction — that whatever illness I may have will be mild and short-lived.

276
I bring myself to fully believe in the power of any medications I am given. I am well aware that, to a great extent, these medicines will generally work as well as I expect them to.

277
I understand that since, with enough positive expectation, even placebos have the power to heal, then certainly a true medication can do the same — and more.

278
I fully expect my body's powerful immune system to destroy any and all diseases that come my way.

279
I know that my thinking literally creates my body and, thus, I can further use the power of my mind to create rapid healing within my body.

280

When I am ill, or recovering from surgery, I spend my time visualizing being well. I *imagine* how good it will feel to be back on my feet. I *feel* how good that will feel!

281

When I am ill or recovering from surgery, I spend my tine visualizing my body working perfectly once again. We are what we think. And I choose to think wellness.

282

I expect to heal quickly.

283

I see myself healing quickly.

284

I feel myself healing quickly.

285

I expect to recover easily.

286

I see myself recovering easily.

287
I feel myself recovering easily.

288
I expect to get back on my feet in no time.

289
I see myself getting back on my feet in no time.

290
I feel myself getting back on my feet in no time.

291
I understand very well that my expectation of a rapid and smooth recovery from illness or surgery is one of the greatest medicines on Earth.

The Power of Affirmation

An affirmation is a positive statement that we repeat many times in order to help bring about a desired result. The power of affirmations is very well-known and very often utilized. People from all professions use affirmations to help bring about financial, or athletic, or professional success. In the realm of health and well-being, our affirmations are even more powerful and effective because they are acting upon our very bodies.

292
When I have an illness, even a serious illness, I use the well-known power of affirmations to help bring about a rapid recovery.

Whenever you are ill or are recovering from injury or surgery, repeat any and all of the following powerful affirmations — often and with conviction:

293
My body is healthy, strong, perfect, and healed.

294
My immune system is killing my disease.

295
My body is healing and growing stronger every day.

296
Every cell in my body vibrates with healthful energy and good health.

297
I am well again — and it feels so good!

298
Every cell in my body is filled with wellness and vitality.

299
I am fully recovered. I heal quickly from illness.

300
I use the power of my mind to heal my body.

301
I have the power to heal quickly from any illness.

302
My mind and body are infinitely more powerful than the collection of viral or bacterial germs occupying it at this moment.

303
Illness ... *be gone!*

304
I feel great! I feel wonderful! I feel strong! I feel better than ever!

305
My immune system is powerful, intelligent, and effective.

306
I don't force my body to heal — I encourage and allow it to heal.

307
I call upon and receive energy from the universe to enter within the energy of my body and remove all of its negative energies, be they sadness, anger, fear, or disease.

308
I am stronger than this illness. I am larger than this illness. I am more powerful than this illness. I am more tenacious than this, or any, illness.

309
I expect — I truly and wholly expect —
to be well soon.

310
My illness is made of *energy*. My mind, body, and spirit are made of *energy* as well — and these are infinitely more powerful than the energy that comprises any illness.

311
I record the above affirmations — repeating them over and over — then I listen to this recording throughout the day.

312
I go one step further by asking family members to record their voices as they repeatedly affirm my healing and recovery.

313

I use affirmations to aid in my healing with the full conviction that they will work, they will work well, and they will work wonders.

The Power of Music

The power of music in helping us to heal and recover more quickly and more completely has been recognized throughout the world for decades. Music lowers a patient's stress levels. It promotes happiness. It stimulates positive brain functioning. It fosters a general sense of well-being. Stroke patients recover faster. And even when under anesthesia, surgery patients exposed to music heal faster and need less pain medication during recovery. When it comes to healing, music is pure magic!

314
I am aware of the incredible power of music in helping to heal from illness or surgery more quickly and completely.

315
I listen to calming, peaceful, soothing, and beautiful music throughout the day during illness or recovery from surgery.

316
I listen to classical music incessantly during times of illness or recovery from surgery for its proven curative power.

317
As I listen, I feel the music's energy bathing my body with its healing power.

318
As I listen, I feel music's energy infusing my body with its incredible healing power.

319
I take advantage of the many multiple hours' long programs on YouTube, or one of the many stations on Pandora or Sirius/XM radio that feature many types of calming, uplifting, inspiring, beautiful, or meditative music, both classical and contemporary.

320
Music heals my body and heals it well.

321
Music invigorates my soul.

322
Music strengthens my immune system.

323
Music reduces my level of pain and anxiety during
illness or recovery from surgery.

324
I enjoy listening to music during procedures and
while receiving infusions to ease
my level of discomfort and anxiety.

325
I understand music's proven power in helping to
restore lost speech resulting from
stroke or brain injury.

326
I recognize the power of music in reducing anxiety
and nausea during chemotherapy.

327
I listen to beautiful, calming music before surgery for
its proven ability to reduce anxiety and lessen
the need for sedatives.

328
I also harness the healing power of music during the
surgery itself, if it is allowed, and especially after
surgery to help me recover faster and with
less need for pain medications.

329
I understand that music decreases my level of anxiety before and after surgery.

330
I intend to take advantage of music's healing powers throughout any illness or surgery I may undergo in the future.

The Power of Prayer

Even amongst the most cynical and least spiritual individuals, the amazing and well-documented power of prayer in healing illness, or in recovery after surgery, can no longer be denied. A person suffering from illness who is prayed for by a "prayer circle" of family and friends will heal or recover faster and with fewer complications than those who are not.

331
I understand that the power of prayer in speeding recovery from either surgery or illness is very well-documented.

332
I enlist family and friends to form a prayer circle on my behalf. I ask them to pray for me — at a preset time each day, if possible — in order to speed my recovery and healing.

333
Given the enormous volume of research proving the power of prayer, I fully believe in its efficacy — and this conviction results in even greater healing for me.

334
I search the Internet for an appropriate healing prayer of my choosing and I offer it to all who will be praying for me.

335
I expect miracles. I understand that to expect miracles is to help bring them about.

336
When I know that loved ones are praying for me, I visualize and feel the power of their collective prayer coursing through my body, filling it with love, giving it strength, and helping me to heal faster.

337
I feel the prayers of my loved ones infusing my being with powerful, healing energy.

338
I feel and visualize the prayers of my loved ones literally pushing disease from my body.

339

I feel the healing energy set forth by my loved ones, in the form of prayer, as it enters my body and soul and gives me the strength to heal, the motivation to fight my illness, and the faith to persevere.

340

When I know that others are praying for me, I fill my mind, body, and soul with gratitude for the powerful, loving, healing energy being sent my way.

341

I visualize the powerful, positive, and healing energy of prayer as pure, white light that surrounds my being with a shield of healing energy.

342

Each time I inhale, I visualize the healing energy of prayer filling me with renewed good health, strength, and vitality.

343

Each time I exhale, I visualize the healing energy of prayer carrying toxins, disease, pain, and negative energy away from my ever-strengthening body.

344

I understand the proven benefits of prayer — and my body, created by my thoughts, grows ever stronger, ever more vital, and ever more healthy.

Be the Perfect Patient

Another powerful tool in our fight against illness is to be the perfect patient, one who fully utilizes all the resources the medical establishment has to offer — from doctors and nurses to medication and counseling — and to fully carry out all instructions given to us.

345
Whenever I am sick or recovering from surgery,
I act as the perfect patient.

346
I do exactly as I am told by my doctors and nurses
and I do so with positivity and kindness.

347
I eat as I am advised to eat.

348
I read any and all literature with
which I am provided.

349
I take all medications I am given exactly as I am directed and with full conviction that they will work and work wonders.

350
I do any exercises that I am advised to do and as often as advised.

351
I do no more and no less than the prescribed amount of physical movement and activity.

352
I do exactly as I am instructed with the understanding and the conviction that it will speed my recovery.

353
To the best of my ability, I am pleasant, polite, and kind to my caregivers. I understand that what goes around, comes around.

354
I am grateful to my doctors and nurses.

355
I send out loving energy to everyone on my medical team, for it will return in kind.

356
I am an inspiration to other patients.

357
I am healthy once again.

358
I am strong once again.

359
I am vital once again.

360
My body is in perfect health once again.

361
I am the perfect patient and I love being alive!

Part Three

AFFIRM YOUR LONGEVITY

"There is a long life ahead of you and it's going to be beautiful as long as you keep loving and hugging each other."

Yoko Ono

Live Long
by Living Well

It goes without saying that, when we treat our bodies right and live by the principles of health and well-being already presented, we will significantly increase our chances of living a very long life.

362

I am made of *energy*. Energy is made of *intelligence* — of *awareness*. I use my thoughts to direct my body to remain youthful and vital regardless of how many years I've been alive.

363

I continually see myself as youthful and vital.

364

I expect to remain youthful and vital regardless of how many years I've been on this earth.

365
My body is made of energy. Energy can neither be created, nor destroyed. It is both timeless and eternal.

366
I continually see and feel my body as being made of creative, ageless energy.

367
I am ageless. There are virtually no cells in my body older than seven years old. If I appear to be "aging," I understand that it is largely because I've expected to do so.

368
Since every cell in my body is made anew within seven years' time, there is no aging other than that which I create with my outmoded thoughts and expectations.

369
My mind has tremendous power in providing me with a very long life.

370
If I choose to direct my thoughts toward longevity, these thoughts will help to bring it about.

371
My thinking can and will keep me alive longer.

372
My thinking can will keep me healthy and fit longer.

373
I think health and well-being — always.

374
I think longevity — always.

375
I desire a very long life.

376
I love the thought of living for a very long time.

377
I am literally what I eat. I keep my body healthy, strong, and youthful by avoiding harmful additives, trans fats, sugar, sodium, chemical additives, and GMOs.

378
I don't glorify the concept of eating solely for pleasure. My life has much to enjoy beyond "dining."

379
I understand that a low-calorie diet is directly linked with longevity.

380
I remain active and energetic regardless of my age. I exercise several times a week and I engage in other vigorous activities every day.

381
I walk as much as possible.

382
I move as much as possible.

383
I stretch as much as possible.

384
I remain productive in some way throughout my later years.

385
I try not to sit for long periods without taking a break by standing and moving around.

386
I greatly prefer the feeling of a strong body to a withered body.

387
I avoid a stressful lifestyle as much as possible. Doing so will add years to my life.

388
I have the freedom to view situations as being either stressful or not stressful. It is my *choice*.

389
I enjoy a healthy, active lifestyle even into my later years.

390
I remain fit for the long haul.

391
I remain active, no matter what my age.

392
I remain positive, no matter how trying certain situations may be.

393
I remain loving, no matter how unloved I may feel.

394
I value each and every one of the friendly and loving connections I have in my life.

395
I work hard at keeping my life full of friends and family.

Live Long
with Positive Expectations

When it comes to health and longevity, *our expectations are king*. To a very large extent, we get the health we expect, we age according to our expectations, and we live as long as we *expect*—that is, to know with certainty and conviction. Our bodies are made from our thinking; thus, our bodies are kept young by our positive expectations.

396
My expectations count for more than genetics.

397
My expectations keep my body young.

398
I expect only the best from my
strong, amazing body.

399
I expect — and choose — to live
for a very long time.

400
I expect — *with conviction* — to live
for a very long time.

401
I expect — *with certainty* — to live
for a very long time.

402
I fully expect to fully enjoy every year
of my long, full life.

403
I expect to remain healthy and strong
as the years move by.

404
I expect to keep my mind healthy and
sharp as the years move by.

405
I expect my body to remain agile and supple.

406
I expect to remain free of disease.

407
I expect to remain active and vital.

408
I expect to remain productive, even after retirement.

409
I expect to remain strong — and I exercise accordingly.

410
I expect — and choose — to remain happy.

411
I expect nothing but the best from my amazing body.

Live Long with Spirituality

The longest-living people are generally quite spiritual. Whether by taking part in organized religion or simply worshipping nature, they operate in a spiritual manner and keep their own spirits bolstered by it.

412
I am a spiritual being.

413
I maintain a spiritual practice throughout my life.

414
Whether in a church, in nature, or in my own private practice, spirituality is an important part of my life.

415
My spiritual practice sustains me.

416
My spiritual practice empowers me.

417
My spirituality helps me to be more loving and thus psychologically, emotionally, and physiologically healthy.

418
I connect deeply with a higher power.

419
I feel the presence of a higher power as I go about my day.

420
I feel protected by a higher power as I go about my day.

421
I enjoy fellowship with others who I meet through my spiritual practice.

422
I invest myself fully in my spiritual practice.

423
My body responds well to my spiritual practices of love, forgiveness, kindness, and hope.

424
I enjoy the feeling of being connected to a power bigger than myself.

425
I understand that my spirituality is one of my life's greatest blessings and one of my lifespan's greatest extenders.

Live Long with a Loving Spirit

Love is the most powerful force in the universe. When we infuse the energy that makes up our bodies with the power of a loving spirit, our bodies grow ever more invincible.

426
I am in love with life.

427
I love all the wonderful people in my life.

428
I love myself.

429
I love my amazing body.

430
I love this beautiful world of ours.

431
I love the splendor and majesty of nature.

432
I love my fellow man.

433
My loving spirit keeps me going.

434
I infuse every cell in my body with the energy of my loving spirit.

435
My heart and mind are filled with loving, healing, sustaining energy.

436
My body is ever renewed by the love I hold in my heart.

437
My heart is renewed with the love I fill it with.

438
I understand that to love much is to live long.

439
I send out vibrations of love to everyone I meet.

440
I am empowered by my loving spirit.

441
My body is strengthened by my loving spirit.

442
My soul is invigorated by my loving spirit.

443
I love the many pleasures with which I fill my day.

444
I love the food I eat.

445
I love seeing and learning new things.

446
I love plants, animals, and beauty.

447
I love being alive.

Live Long
by Remaining Unbuggable

The benefits of remaining unbuggable through life's trials and tribulations are very well-documented. It has often been regarded as a primary shared characteristic of centenarians: the ability to remain level-headed and at peace through just about any trying situation. Living by this practice not only helps to extend our lifespan — it improves our quality of life as well.

448
I understand and value the importance of remaining unbuggable as a means of increasing my lifespan.

449
I am emotionally strong.

450
I am resilient.

451
I am in control.

452
I am cool-headed in all situations.

453
I am larger than any adversity that may come my way.

454
No matter what life throws at me, I shake it off and carry on.

455
I practice the life-enhancing art of *detachment*.

456
I remain steady, calm, unruffled, and strong in the face of, adversity, loss, or setback.

457
I maintain equanimity — calm imperturbability — in all situations.

458
I understand that life contains struggle and I meet each struggle head on.

459
No matter what, I will prevail over loss or setback.

460
I shrug off anything life throws at me.

461
I am unshakable.

462
I am unbreakable.

463
I am unbeatable.

464
I am unstoppable.

465
I am powerful.

466
I am resilient.

467
I am bigger than my problems.

468
I am too large for worry.

469
I am too happy for despair.

470
I live long and prosper through the practice of remaining supremely unbuggable.

Live Long by Shooting For 100

You have nothing to lose and so much to gain by fully expecting, anticipating, and working toward achieving a lifespan of more than 100 years. Take on this quest enthusiastically, joyfully, and confidently. Again, you have nothing to lose and everything to gain. Life is, indeed, precious! Live as long a life as you possibly can. The *quantity* of years you ultimately live may not seem as important as the *quality* of those years, but just remember: the more years you live the more opportunities you'll have for enjoying quality years full of many, many beautiful moments!

471
As far as I'm concerned, I am going to live beyond 100 years of age or die trying!

472
For me, it's 100-plus or bust.

473
100! love that number and think of it often.

474
100 years and more… Why not *try*?

475
100 years and beyond… Why not *me*?

476
Thousands of people each year make it beyond 100. Why *not* me?

477
I understand that one reason most people don't make it to 100 is because they don't think it's possible for them and so they don't even try. I am definitely not one of them!

478
So many people believe that longevity is predetermined by luck or fate or genetics. I know better.

479
There is so much that I want to experience and do in my life. I will need *at least* 100 years to do it all!

480
I am too busy living and loving life to grow old.

481
Rocking chairs are not my style.

482
I have no intention of "slowing down."

483
I have over 100 years' worth of goals
that I intend to pursue.

484
The life in my years? The years in my life?
I choose *both*.

485
I have nothing to lose and much to gain by setting
my intention to live beyond
the century mark.

486
I have a strong survival instinct and I want to live and
experience as much as I can in this lifetime.

487
I am not going anywhere until I do all
that I want to do.

488
The Indian sage Shankara once said that "people grow old and die because they see other people grow old and die." I have no intention of causing myself to age simply by subconsciously programming myself to do so.

489
There are nearly 320,000 centenarians in the world and that number is expected to multiply eightfold by 2050. Though I am in no rush to get there, I intend to be one of them.

490
I have absolutely nothing to lose by shooting for 100 and more.

491
I can make it past 100.

492
I expect to live beyond 100.

493
I will see beyond my 100th birthday.

494
I look forward to living beyond 100 in perfect health.

495
So many people make it past 100 ... some even venture beyond 110. Why ... not ... me?

496
I am forever healthy.

497
I am forever strong.

498
I am forever vital.

499
My body is forever in perfect health.

500
I love, love, *love* being alive!

Take these affirmations to heart. Read these affirmations often. Recite your favorites every day. Write down your favorites on index cards and carry them with you. Review them regularly. More important: Practice what they preach. Live by them. Teach them to others. And make a plan to review them on your 100th birthday!

Most of all, enjoy a rich, rewarding, happy, healthy, and very long life!

About the Author

Stan Munslow is an author and educator. He has spent the past twenty years researching aging, longevity, and quantum healing and, at 58 years old, he has never been hospitalized, never had surgery and, other than a touch of flu thirteen years ago and a handful of colds, he has never been sick. His morning workout routine includes two hundred nonstop pushups and he moves through his day with more vim and vigor than most teenagers. He lives in Rhode Island with his wife and his Maltese pooch, Boo.

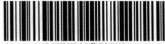

Made in the USA
Columbia, SC
25 April 2018